Juicing For Osteoporosis

26 Juicing Recipes To Develop & Maintain Healthy Bones in Women

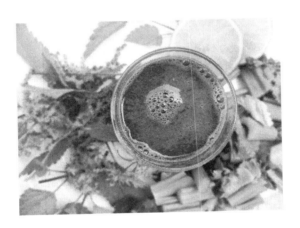

Les S. Rosado

Copyright © [2023] by Les S. Rosado.

More Books By This Author

Surviving Osteoporosis Cookbook
30 Anti-Inflammatory Herbal Tinctures For
Cancer Treatment
The Vegan Wild Mushrooms Cookbook

Table of Contents

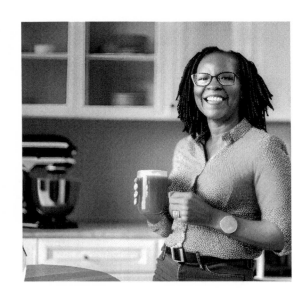

Introduction

In the quiet corners of the modern world, a silent epidemic looms, affecting millions of women. Osteoporosis, the thief of strength and mobility, strikes at the very foundation of our skeletal system. But fear not, for within these pages lies a delicious remedy, a vibrant elixir that holds the power to fortify and rejuvenate your bones. Welcome to *"Juicing for Osteoporosis: 26 Juicing Recipes to Develop & Maintain Healthy Bones in Women,"* where nature's bounty intertwines with cutting-edge nutrition. Join us on a transformative journey through the vibrant world of juicing, as we unveil a treasure trove of liquid vitality that will nourish your bones from within. Immerse yourself in a symphony of colors, flavors, and nutrients, as we present 25 meticulously crafted juicing recipes, each designed to optimize bone health and defy the grasp of osteoporosis. Unleash the healing power of fruits, vegetables, and herbs, and embark on a path towards strong, resilient bones. Let the kaleidoscope of flavors guide you as we sip our way to a future where osteoporosis is nothing but a distant memory.

In these pages, you will unlock the alchemical secrets that lie within every juicing recipe. Discover the transformative effects of nature's potent ingredients, carefully selected to deliver a symphony of vitamins, minerals, and antioxidants directly to your bones. From the refreshing citrus burst of orange and grapefruit to the earthy embrace of kale and spinach, each recipe is a harmonious blend of flavors designed to tantalize your taste buds while bolstering your skeletal strength. With every sip, you'll feel the surge of life-giving nutrients infuse your body, nourishing your bones with the essential elements they crave.

The journey to healthier bones begins now!

26 Juicing Recipes For Strong & Healthy Bones

These are some of the best juicing recipes for preventing and managing osteoporosis in women. Each recipe includes an ingredients list, preparation time, preparation method, and nutritional value per serving. Enjoy each of these delicious and nutritious juicing recipes to support you on your quest to build strong and healthy bones!

1. Green Goddess Juice

Preparation time: 10 minutes
Ingredients:
- 1 cup kale
- 1 cup spinach
- 1 cucumber
- 1 apple
- 1 lemon
- 1 inch piece of ginger
- ½ cup water

Preparation method:
1. Wash all of the ingredients.
2. Add all of the ingredients to a juicer and juice.
3. Fill a glass with the juice and enjoy.

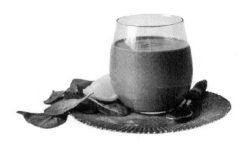

2. Orange Dream Juice

Preparation time: 10 minutes
Ingredients:
- 2 oranges
- 1 carrot
- 1 apple
- ½ cucumber
- 1 inch piece of ginger
- ½ cup water

Preparation method:
1. Wash all of the ingredients.
2. Add all of the ingredients to a juicer and juice.
3. Fill a glass with the juice and enjoy.

3. Berry Blast Juice

Preparation time: 10 minutes
Ingredients:
- 1 cup blueberries
- 1 cup raspberries
- 1 cup strawberries
- 1 banana
- ½ cucumber
- ½ cup water

Preparation method:

1. Wash all of the ingredients.
2. Add all of the ingredients to a juicer and juice.
3. Fill a glass with the juice and enjoy.

4. Tropical Delight Juice

Preparation time: 10 minutes
Ingredients:

- 1 pineapple
- 1 mango
- 1 banana
- ½ cucumber
- ½ cup of water

Preparation method:
1. Wash all of the ingredients.
2. Add all of the ingredients to a juicer and juice.
3. Fill a glass with the juice and enjoy.

5. Beetroot Booster Juice

Preparation time: 10 minutes

Ingredients:

- 1 beetroot
- 1 apple
- 1 carrot
- ½ cucumber
- 1 inch piece of ginger
- ½ cup water

Preparation method:

1. Wash all of the ingredients.
2. Peel the beetroot.
3. Add all of the ingredients to a juicer and juice.
4. Fill a glass with the juice and enjoy.

6. Recipe: Green Calcium Boost

Preparation time: 10 minutes
Ingredients:
- 2 cups kale
- 1 cup spinach
- 1 cucumber
- 2 celery stalks
- 1 green apple
- 1 lemon (juiced)

Preparation method:
1. Juice all the ingredients together.
2. Serve immediately.

7. Recipe: Berry Bone Strength

Preparation Time: 5 minutes
Ingredients:
- 1 cup strawberries
- 1 cup blueberries
- 1 cup raspberries
- 1 cup almond milk

- 1 tablespoon chia seeds

Preparation method:
1. Blend the ingredients thoroughly until smooth.
2. Serve chilled.

8. Tropical Bone Booster

Preparation time: 5 minutes
Ingredients:
- 1 cup pineapple
- 1 orange
- 1 banana
- 1 cup coconut water
- 1 tablespoon flax seeds

Preparation method:
1. Juice the pineapple, orange, and banana.
2. Mix the juice with coconut water and blend in the flaxseeds.
3. Serve chilled.

9. Almond-Broccoli Blend

Preparation time: 5 minutes
Ingredients:

- 1 cup broccoli florets
- 1 cup almond milk
- 1 tablespoon almond butter
- 1 teaspoon honey

Preparation method:

1. Steam the broccoli until tender.
2. Blend the steamed broccoli with almond milk, almond butter, and honey until smooth.
3. Serve chilled.

10. Recipe: Citrus Kale Crush

Preparation time: 7 minutes
Ingredients:

- 2 oranges
- 2 cups kale
- 1 carrot
- 1-inch ginger root

Preparation method:
1. Juice the oranges, kale, carrot, and ginger.
2. Mix well and serve immediately.

11. Beetroot-Berry Blast

Preparation time: 6 minutes
Ingredients:
- 1 small beetroot
- Mixed berries (strawberries, blueberries, raspberries) 1 cup
- 1 cup coconut water
- 1 tablespoon honey

Preparation method:
1. Juice the beetroot and berries.
2. Mix the juice with coconut water and honey.
3. Serve chilled.

12. Spinach-Banana Delight

Preparation time: 5 minutes
Ingredients:
- 2 cups spinach
- 2 bananas
- 1 cup almond milk
- 1 tablespoon almond butter

Preparation method:
1. Blend the spinach, bananas, almond milk, and almond butter until smooth.
2. Serve immediately.

13. Carrot-Orange Nourisher

Preparation time: 5 minutes
Ingredients:
- 4 carrots
- 2 oranges
- 1-inch turmeric root
- 1 tablespoon hon

Preparation method:
1. Juice the carrots, oranges, and turmeric.
2. Stir in honey and serve immediately.

14. Creamy Avocado Kale

Preparation time: 7 minutes
Ingredients:

- 2 cups kale
- 1 avocado
- 1 green apple
- 1 cup almond milk
- Juice of 1 lime

Preparation method:

1. Blend the kale, avocado, green apple, almond milk, and lime juice until creamy.
2. Serve chilled.

15. Pineapple-Spinach Refresher

Preparation time: 6 minutes
Ingredients:

- 1 cup spinach
- 1 cup pineapple chunks
- 1 cucumber
- 1 lime (juiced)
- 1 tablespoon fresh mint leaves

Preparation method:
1. Juice the spinach, pineapple, cucumber, and lime juice.
2. Blend in fresh mint leaves.
3. Serve over ice.

16. Blueberry - Almond Zest

Preparation time: 5 minutes
Ingredients:
- 1 cup blueberries
- 1 cup almond milk
- 1 tablespoon almond butter
- 1 tablespoon flax seeds

Preparation method:
1. Blend the blueberries, almond milk, almond butter, and flaxseeds until smooth.
2. Serve chilled.

17. Kiwi-Cucumber Vitality

Preparation time: 5 minutes
Ingredients:
- 2 kiwis
- 1 cucumber
- 1 cup coconut water
- 1 tablespoon honey

Preparation method:
1. Juice the kiwis and cucumber.
2. Mix the juice with coconut water and honey.
3. Serve chilled.

18. Ginger-Turmeric Elixir

Preparation time: 5 minutes
Ingredients:
- 1-inch ginger root
- 1-inch turmeric root
- 2 oranges
- 1 lemon (juiced)
- 1 tablespoon honey

Preparation method:
1. Juice the ginger, turmeric, oranges, and lemon juice.
2. Stir in honey and serve immediately.

19. Mango-Papaya Punch

Preparation time: 6 minutes
Ingredients:
- 1 mango
- 1 papaya
- 1 orange
- 1 cup coconut water

Preparation method:
1. Juice the mango, papaya, and orange.
2. Mix the juice with coconut water.
3. Serve chilled.

20. Basil-Strawberry Refresher

Preparation time: 5 minutes
Ingredients:
- 1 cup strawberries
- 1 cup coconut water
- 1 tablespoon fresh basil leaves
- 1 tablespoon lime juice

Preparation method:
1. Blend the strawberries, coconut water, basil leaves, and lime juice until smooth.
2. Serve chilled.

21. Spinach - Mango Delight

Preparation time: 5 minutes
Ingredients:
- 2 cups spinach
- 1 mango
- 1 banana
- 1 cup almond milk

Preparation method:
1. Blend the spinach, mango, banana, and almond milk until smooth.
2. Serve immediately.

22. Cranberry - Beet Boost

Preparation time: 6 minutes
Ingredients:
- 1 cup cranberries
- 1 small beetroot
- 1 green apple
- 1 lemon (juiced)
- 1 tablespoon honey

Preparation method:
1. Juice the cranberries, beetroot, green apple, and lemon juice.
2. Stir in honey and serve immediately.

23. Pomegranate - Kale Elixir

Preparation time: 8 minutes
Ingredients:
- 1 cup pomegranate seeds
- 2 cups kale
- 1 cucumber
- 1 tablespoon chia seeds
- 1 tablespoon honey

Preparation method:
1. Juice the pomegranate seeds, kale, and cucumber.
2. Mix in chia seeds and honey.
3. Serve chilled.

24. Orange - Carrot Twist

Preparation time: 5 minutes
Ingredients:
- 2 oranges
- 2 carrots
- 1-inch ginger root
- 1 tablespoon honey

Preparation method:
1. Juice the oranges, carrots, and ginger.
2. Stir in honey and serve immediately.

25. Minty Melon Refresher

Preparation time: 5 minutes
Ingredients:
- 2 cups watermelon
- 1 cup honeydew melon
- 1 tablespoon fresh mint leaves
- Juice of 1 lime

Preparation method:
1. Blend the watermelon, honeydew melon, mint leaves, and lime juice until smooth.
2. Serve chilled.

26.Turmeric-Spinach Powerhouse

Preparation time: 7 minutes
Ingredients:
- 2 cups spinach
- 1 cucumber
- 1 green apple
- 1-inch turmeric root
- 1 lemon (juiced)
- 1 tablespoon coconut oil

Preparation method:
1. Juice the spinach, cucumber, green apple, and turmeric.
2. Pour in the lemon juice and coconut oil and mix.
3. Serve chilled.

Conclusion

As we come to the end of our juicing journey for healthy bones, we hope you have found inspiration, knowledge, and a renewed sense of empowerment. We have explored the remarkable healing potential of fruits, vegetables, and herbs, harnessing their inherent power to nourish and protect our skeletal system. Through these 26 carefully crafted juicing recipes, you have discovered a symphony of flavors and nutrients that can transform your bone health.

But remember, this book is only the beginning. The recipes within are gateways to a broader world of wellness. Continue to explore and experiment with ingredients, tailoring the recipes to suit your individual tastes and needs. Embrace the concept of juicing as a lifelong commitment to your bone health.

Together, let us raise a glass to the remarkable strength and resilience of the female body. May your bones remain robust and unyielding, a testament to the vitality within. Cheers to a future where osteoporosis is a distant memory, and vibrant, healthy bones become a lifelong companion.

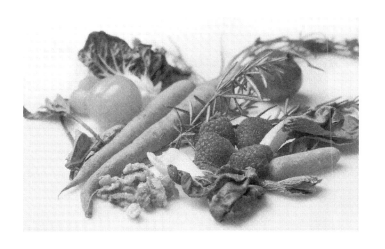

Made in United States
Troutdale, OR
10/15/2024